# A Great Day in Ghana

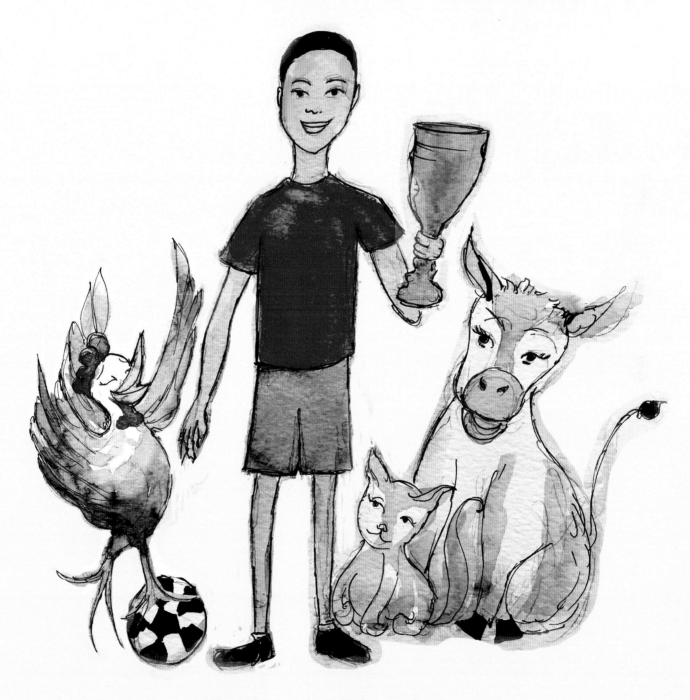

## By David Messick
## Illustrated by Cory Steiger

*Dedicated to Coach Steve Shaw, "Moses," and all of our friends in Ghana and America who made this story possible.*

A Great Day in Ghana
By David Messick
Illustrated by Cory Steiger

© Copyright 2024 / All Rights Reserved
Text and Original Photos: David Messick
Illustrations: Cory Steiger

First Printing / Printed in the USA

ISBN: 979-8-9893939-1-6

Rainbow Puppet Publications
18 Easthill Court,
Hampton, Virginia 23664
Rainbow Puppet Productions is a non-profit,
educational entertainment company

www.rainbowpuppets.com

Designed by Virginia Gabriele

Rainbow Puppeteers include James Cooper, Wesley Huff, Alyssa Jones,
David and Joshua Messick

Thanks to
Traci Massie, Erin Matteson, Curtis Johnson and Sentara Health Plans,
Tony Gabriele, David & Stephanie Messick, Marcy Messick,
Nancy Kent Swilley, and Rose West

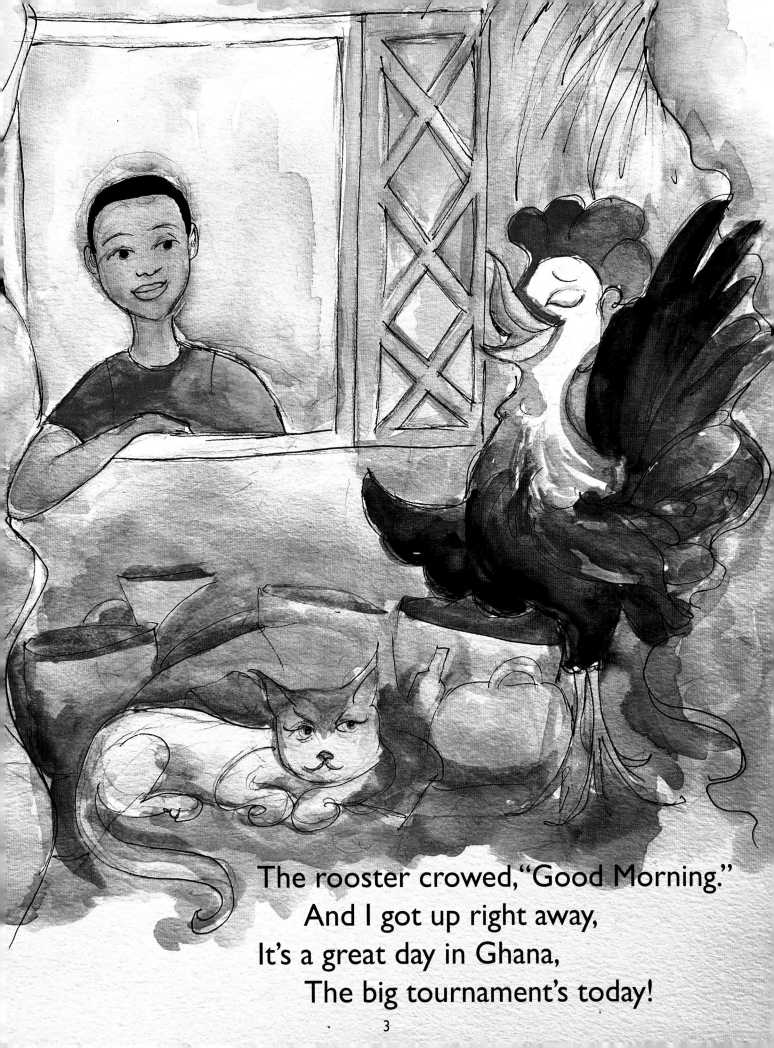

The rooster crowed, "Good Morning."
And I got up right away,
It's a great day in Ghana,
The big tournament's today!

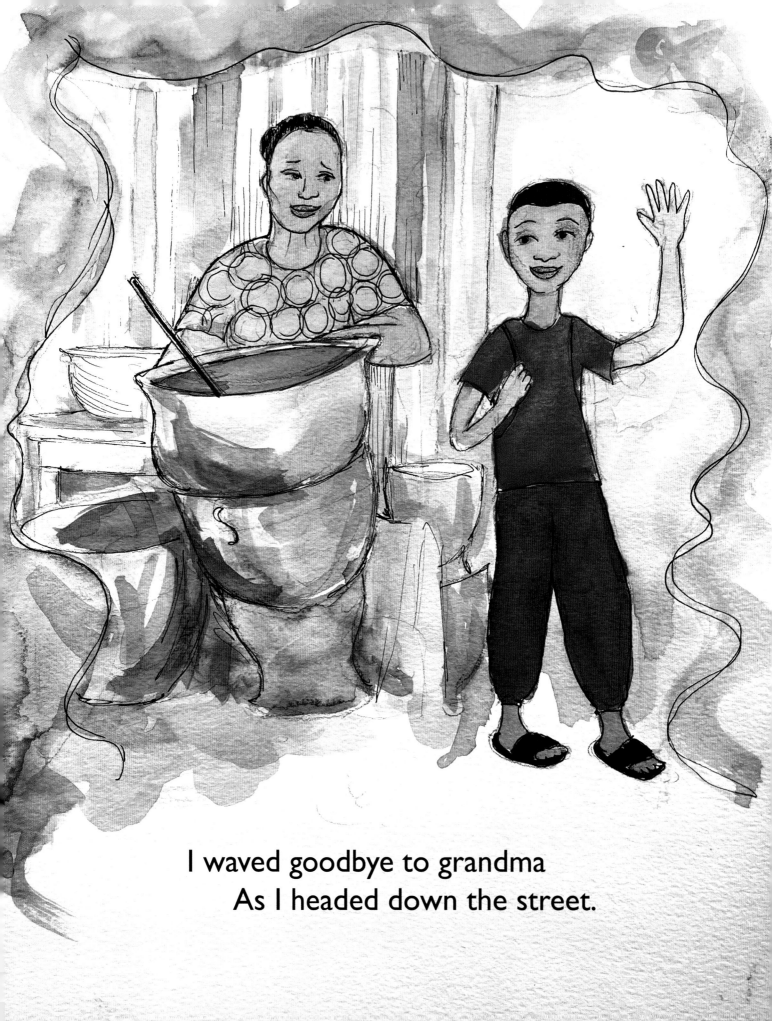

I waved goodbye to grandma
As I headed down the street.

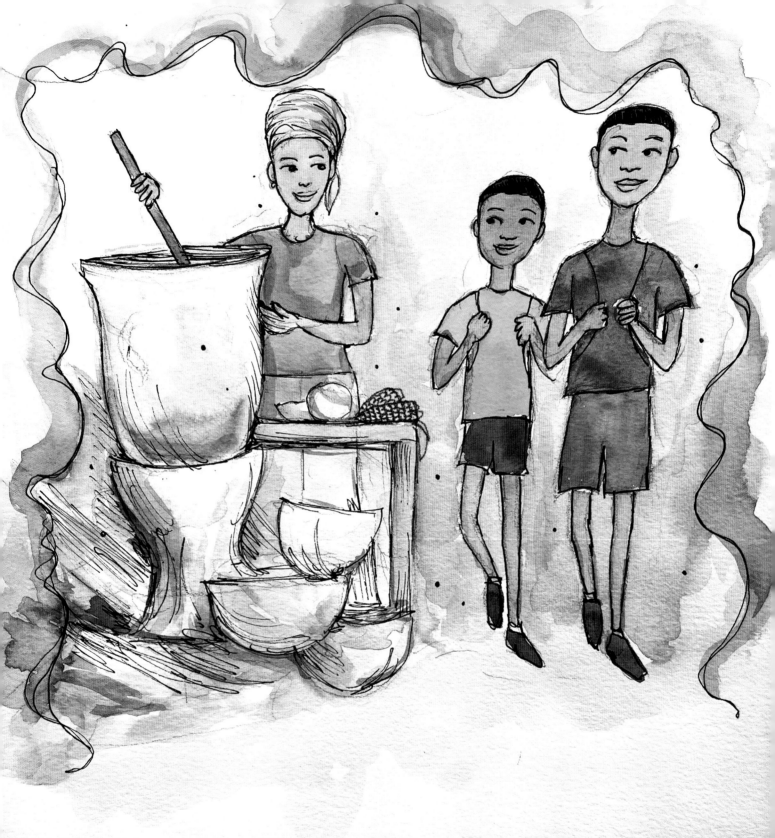

And even "Mama's" yummy corn
Could not slow down my feet.

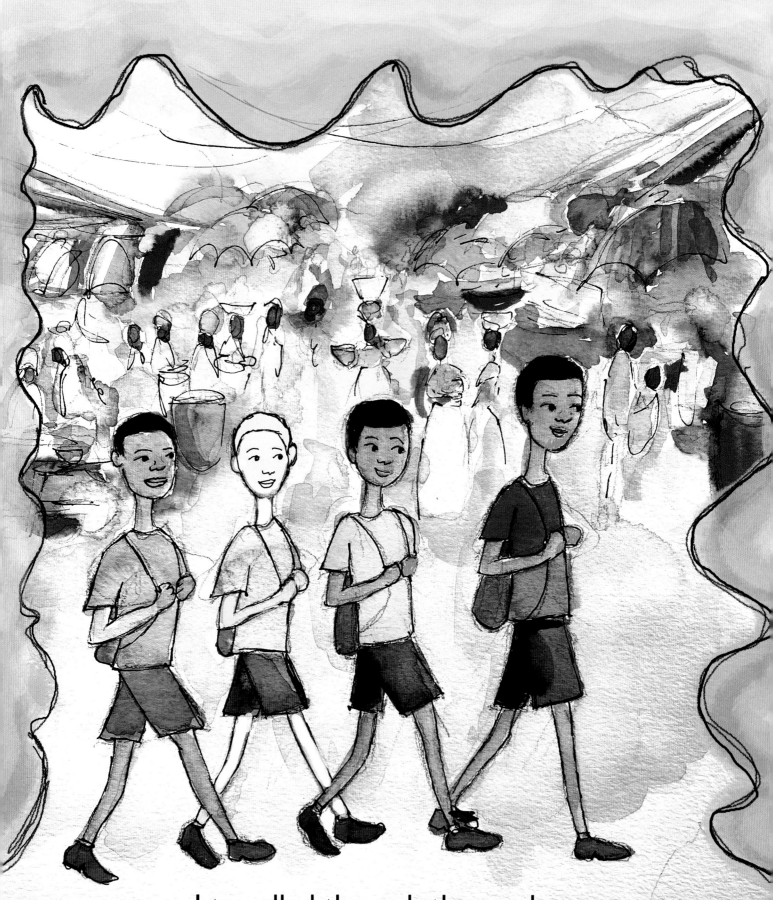

I travelled through the market
As I gathered up my friends.

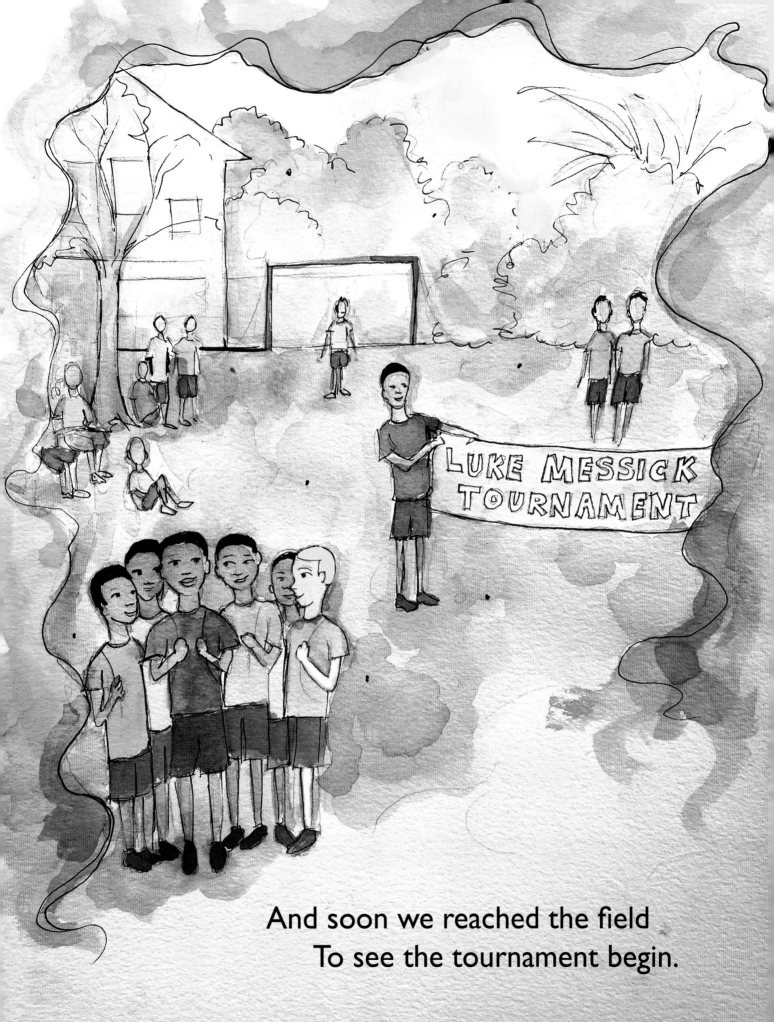

And soon we reached the field
To see the tournament begin.

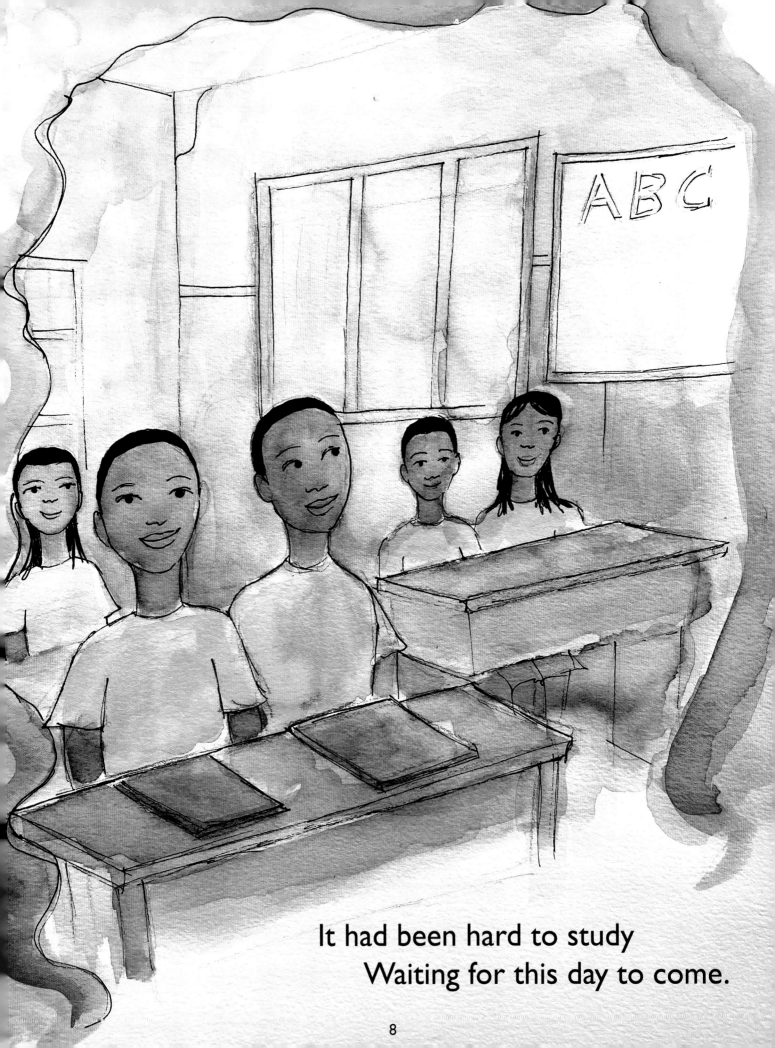

It had been hard to study
Waiting for this day to come.

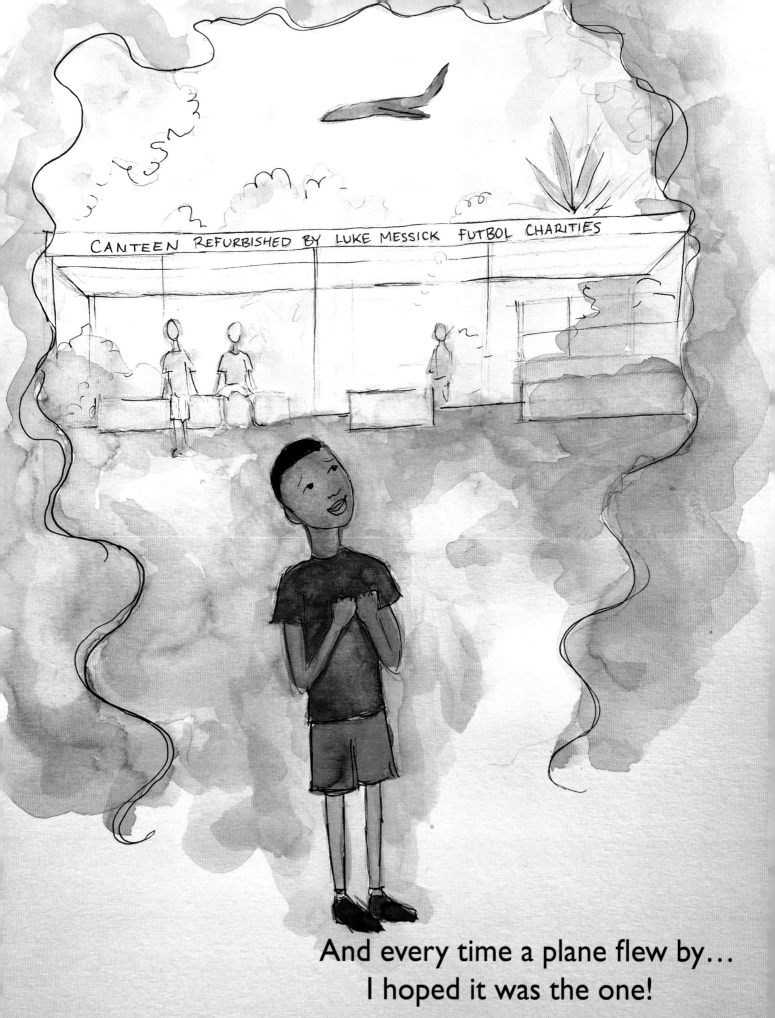

And every time a plane flew by…
I hoped it was the one!

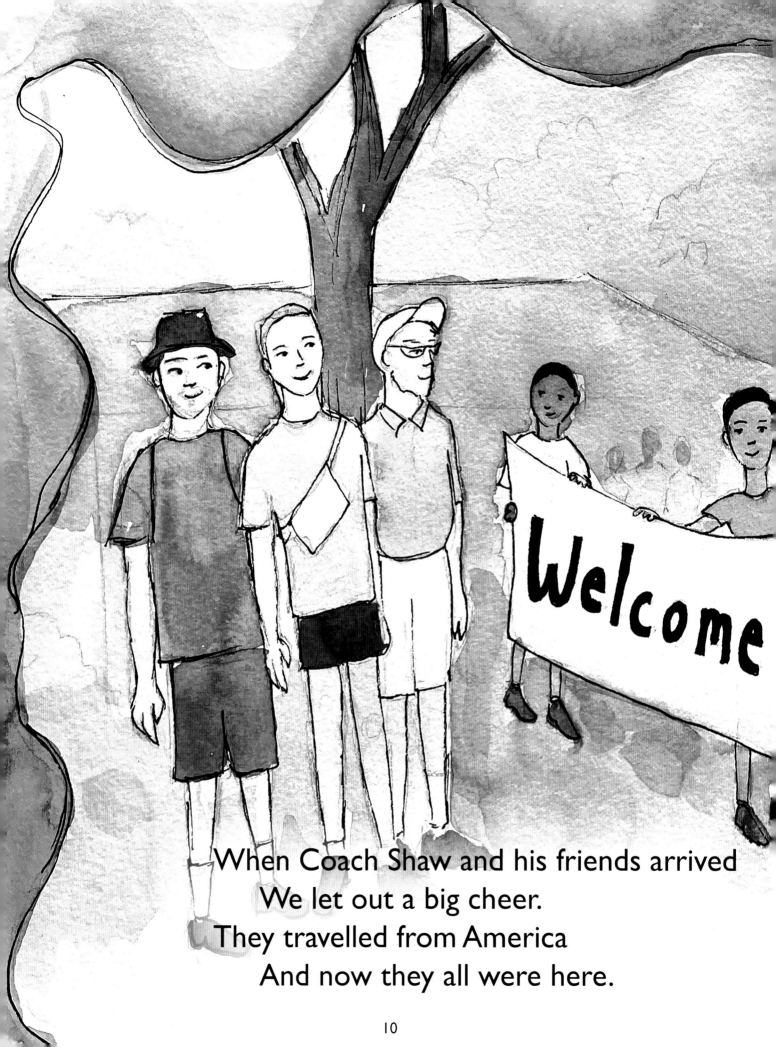

When Coach Shaw and his friends arrived
We let out a big cheer.
They travelled from America
And now they all were here.

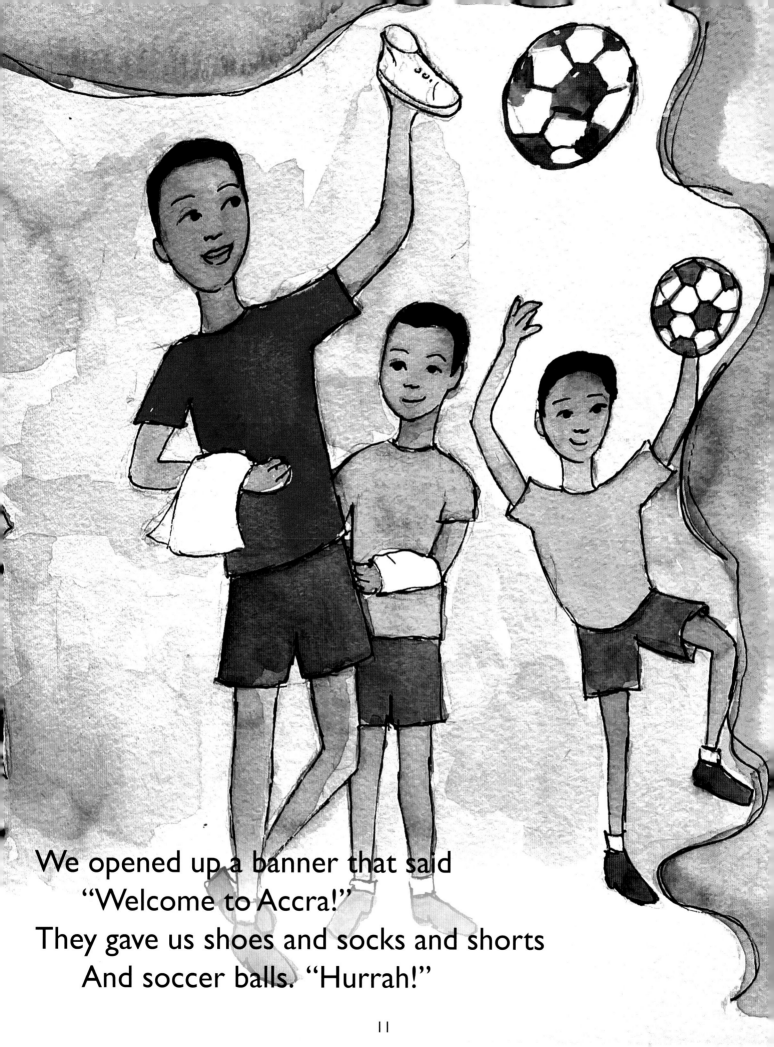

We opened up a banner that said
   "Welcome to Accra!"
They gave us shoes and socks and shorts
   And soccer balls. "Hurrah!"

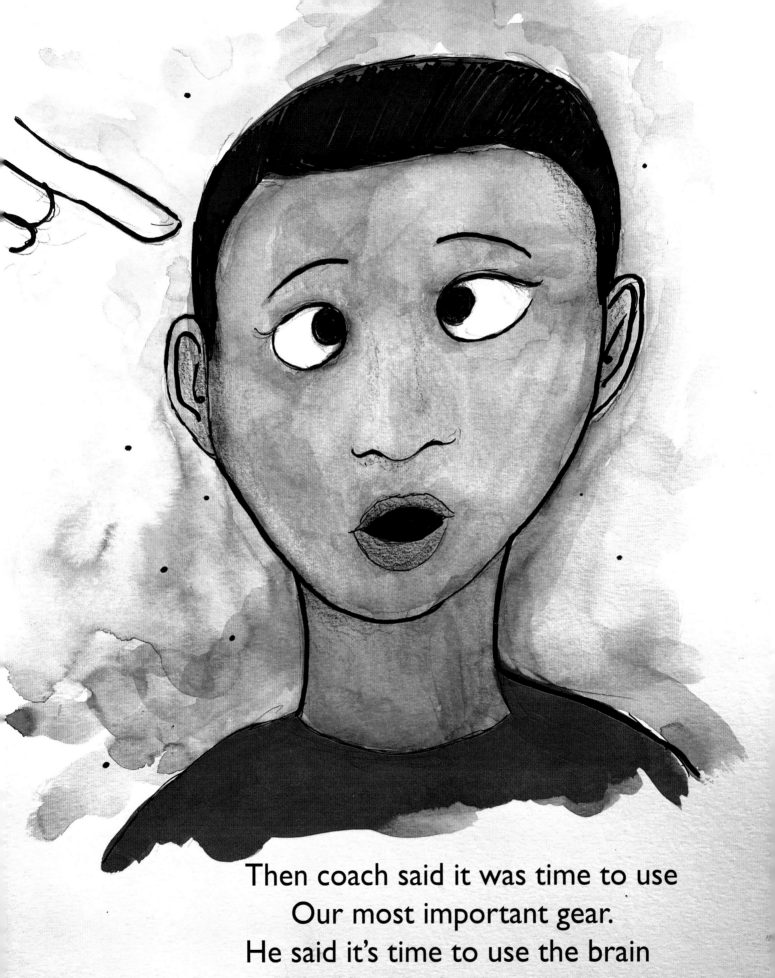

Then coach said it was time to use
Our most important gear.
He said it's time to use the brain
That's right between our ears.

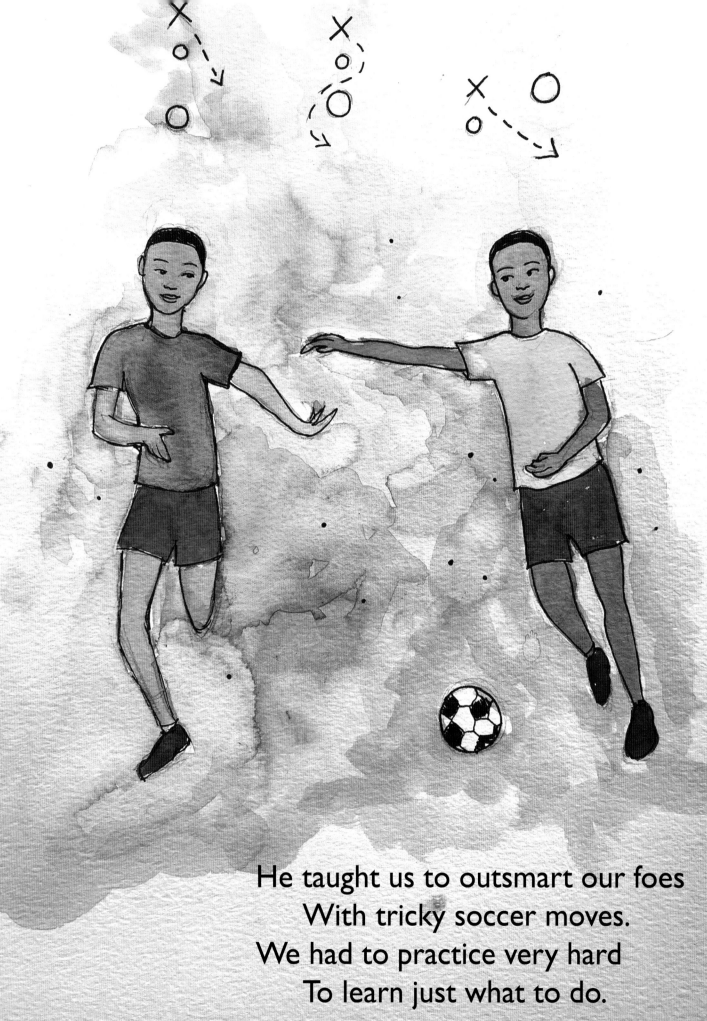

He taught us to outsmart our foes
With tricky soccer moves.
We had to practice very hard
To learn just what to do.

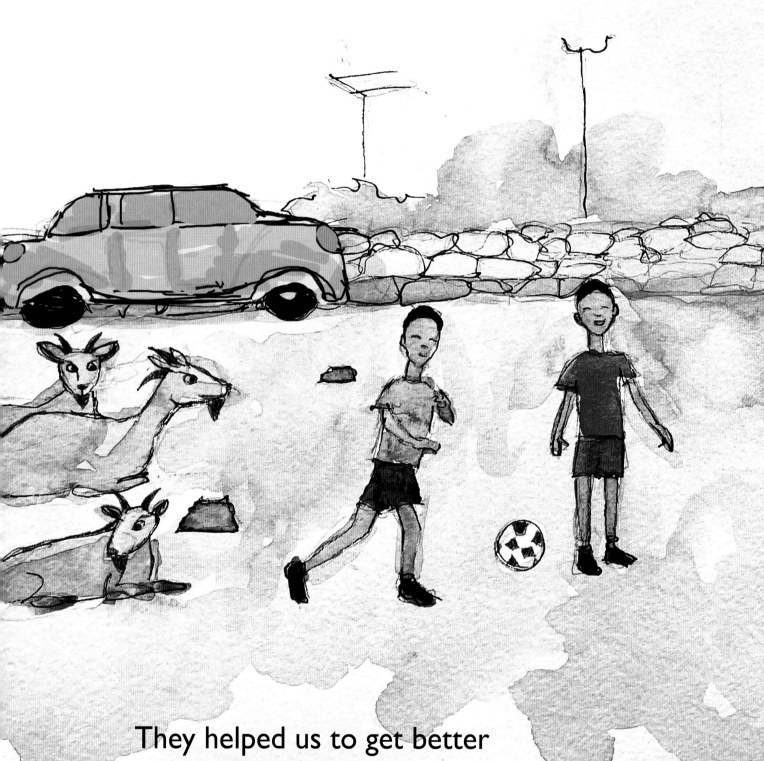

They helped us to get better
As we practiced every day.
But sometimes cars and goats and rocks
And bulls got in the way!

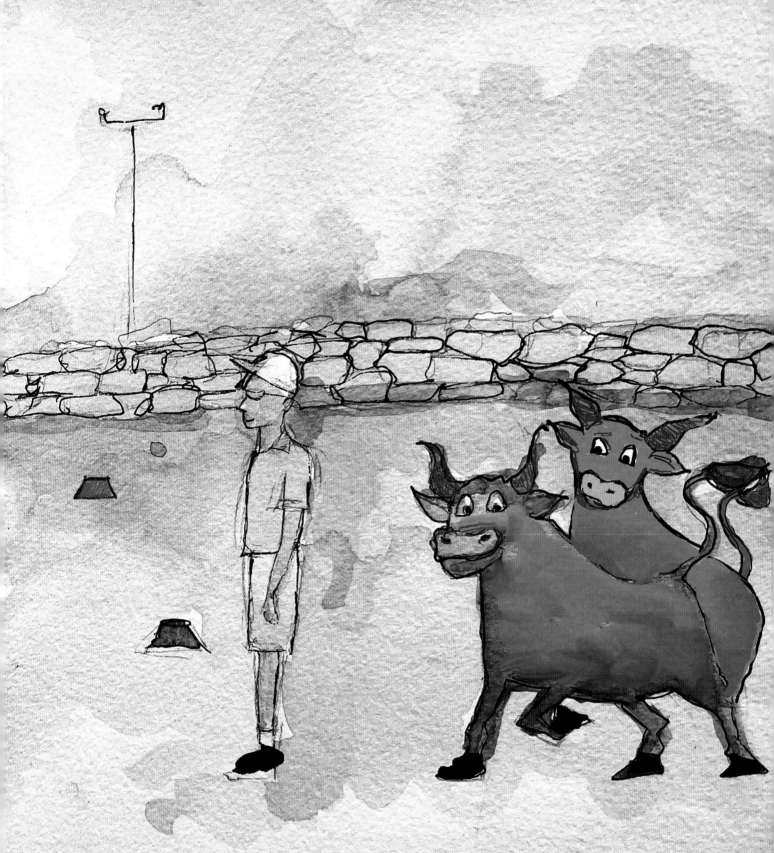

The coach just kept on coaching,
Acting like he didn't care.
"If you can win on this field,
You can win most anywhere!"

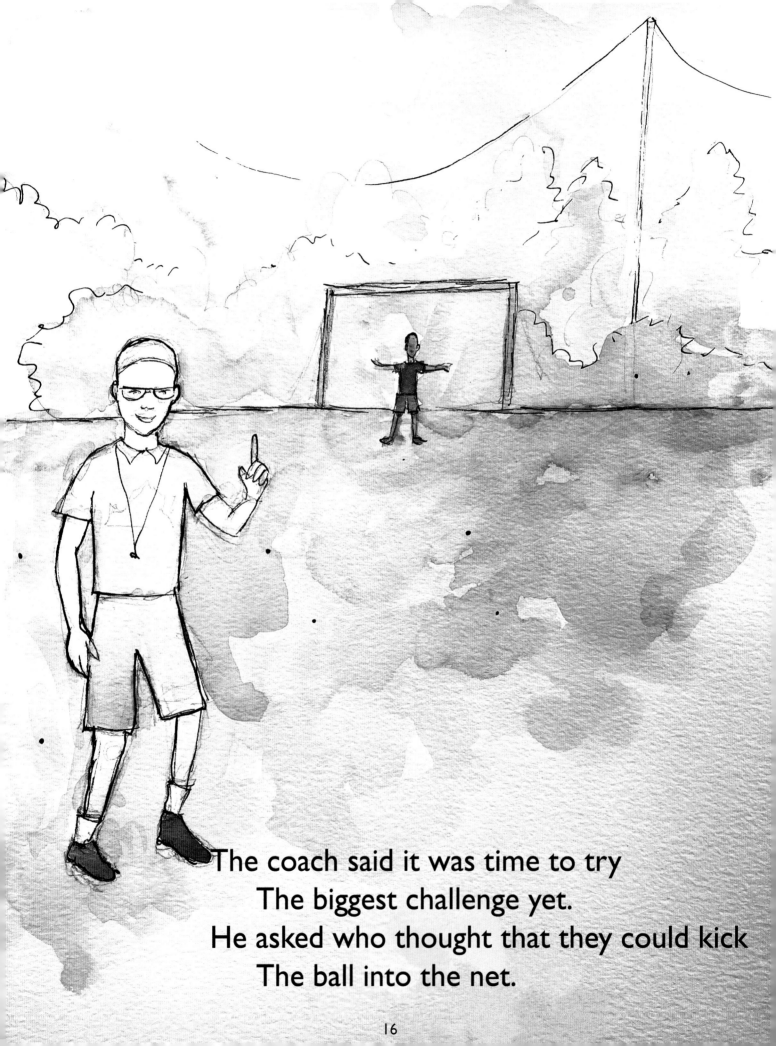

The coach said it was time to try
The biggest challenge yet.
He asked who thought that they could kick
The ball into the net.

The field got really quiet
　　When I slowly raised my hand.
I took a breath and then I told him,
　　"I believe I can!"

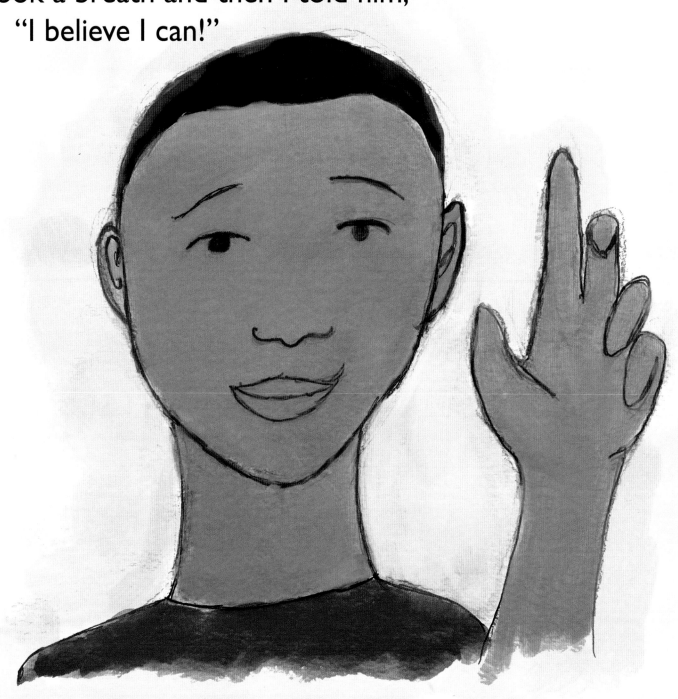

Then coach told me a secret
　　That he said was "power-packed."
He said he learned it long ago,
　　He called it, "Look, Plan, Act."

"First you have to LOOK
To see the problems you must solve.

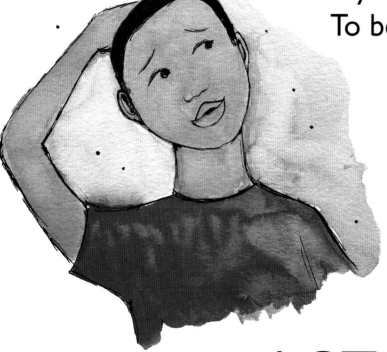

Then you make a PLAN
To beat the challenges involved.

Now, you're set to ACT
And make the problems go away.

And if it comes together you are sure to win the day."

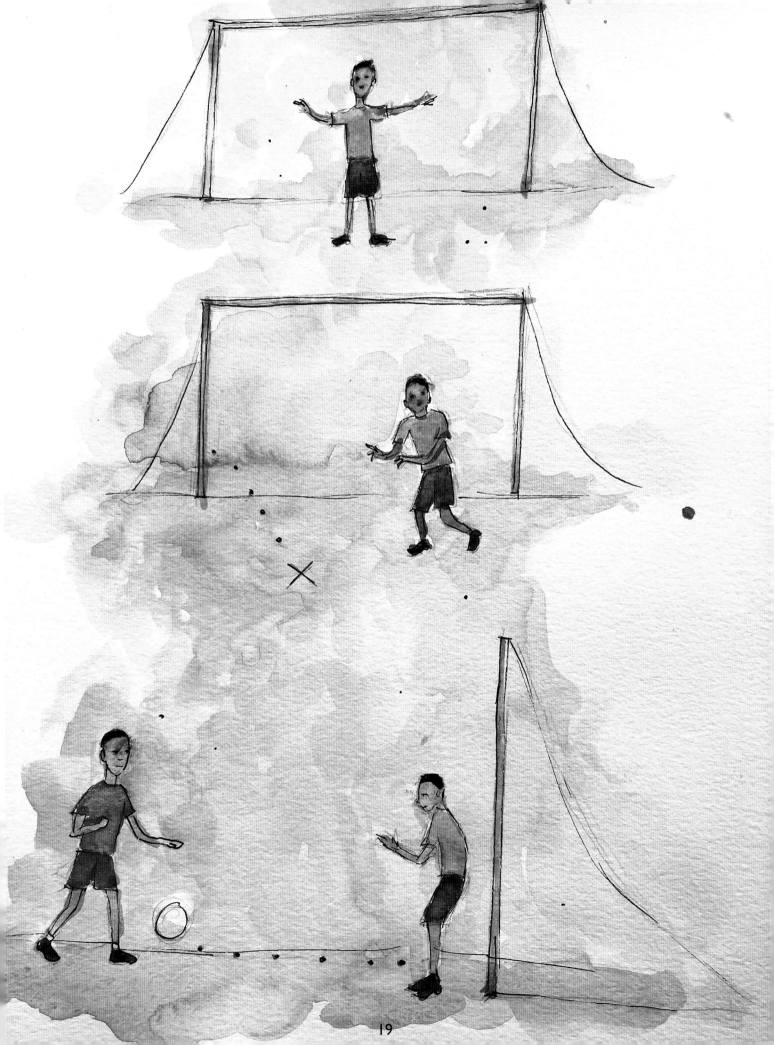

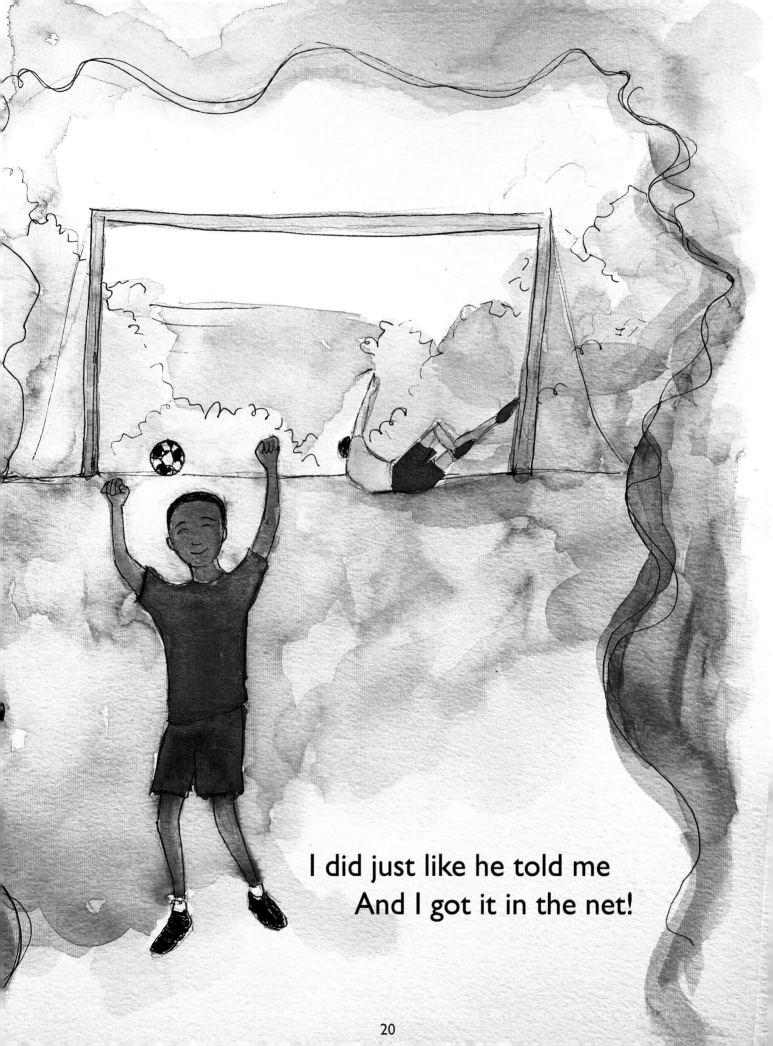

I did just like he told me
And I got it in the net!

Then coach said, "Now we're ready
For the three-game tournament."

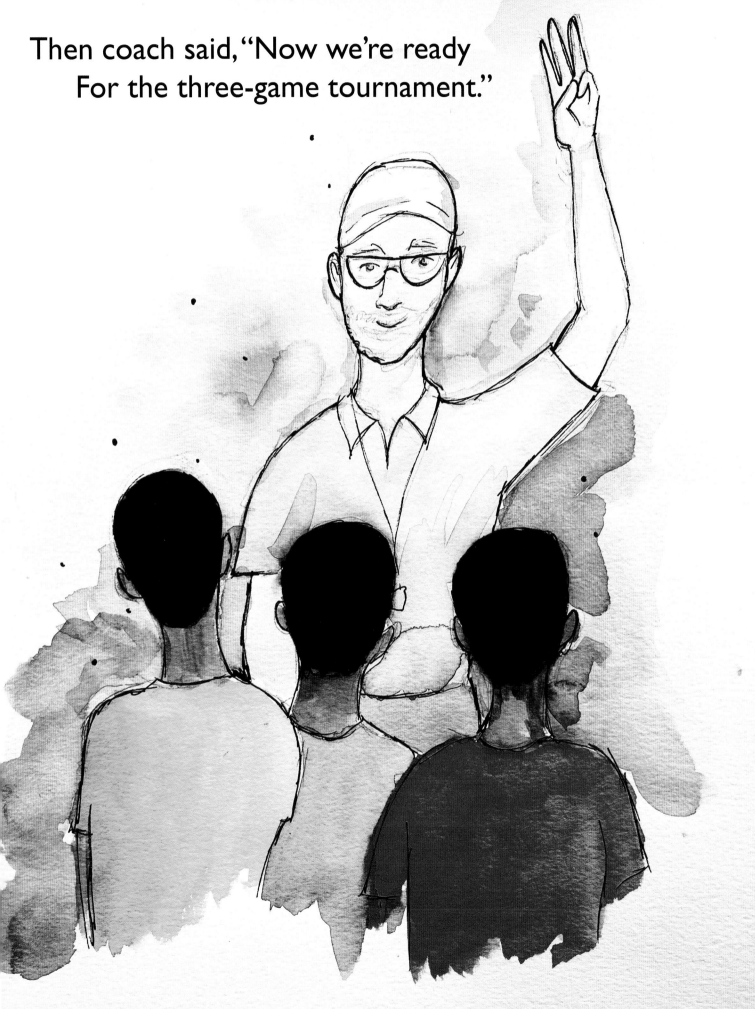

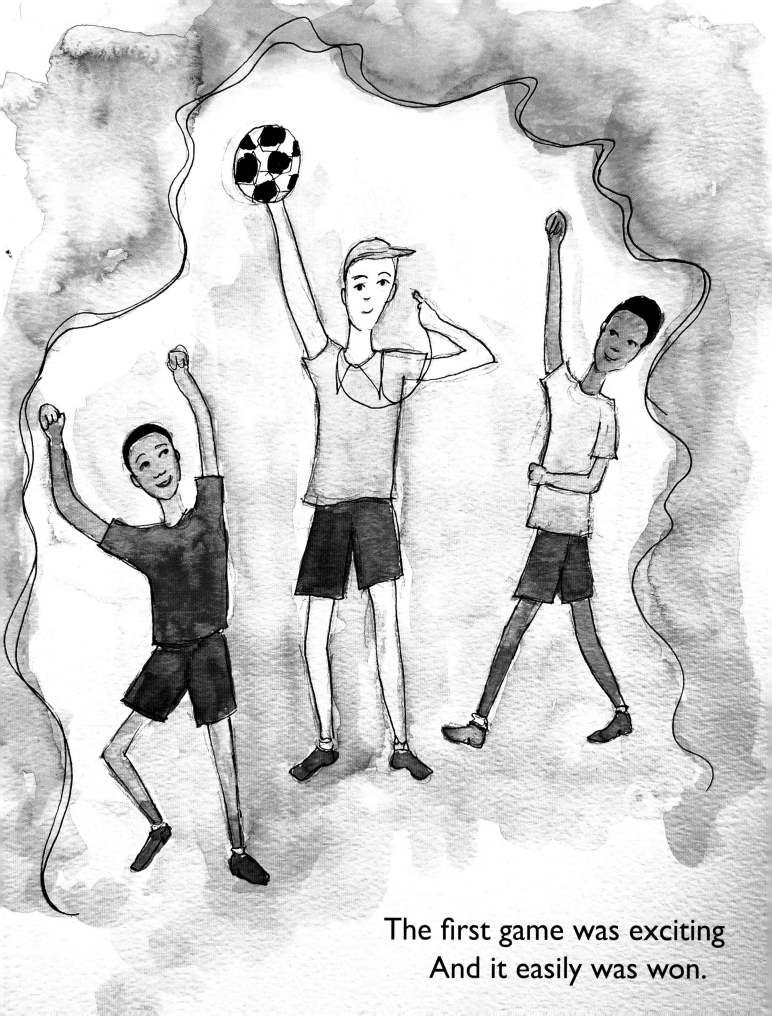

The first game was exciting
And it easily was won.

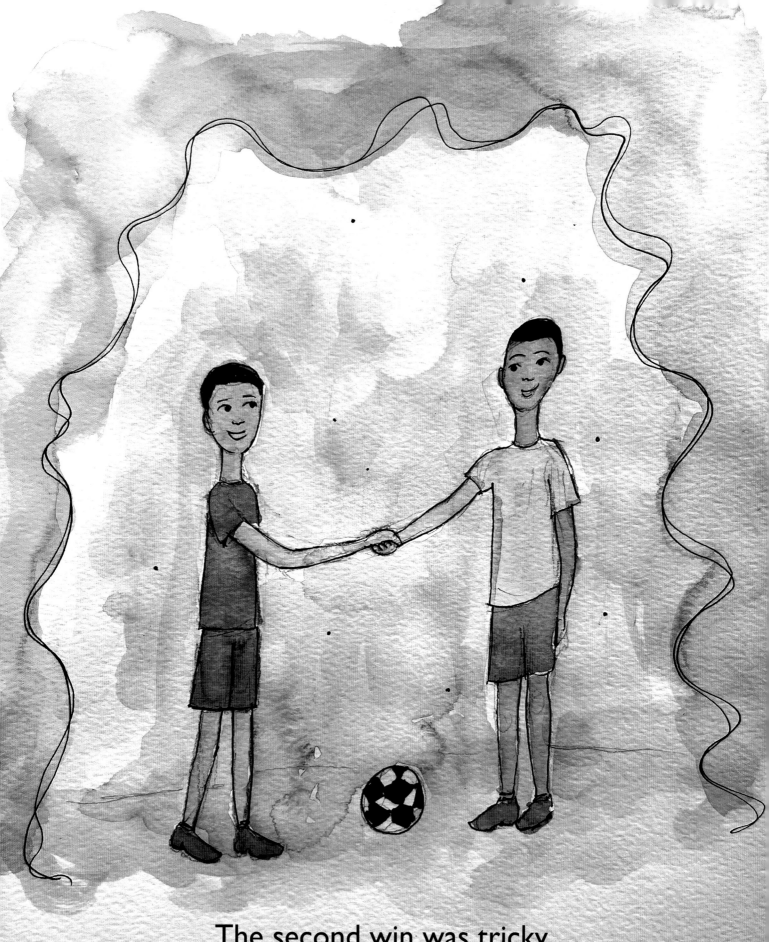

The second win was tricky
But we had a lot of fun.

We took a break and got to eat
    Delicious jollof rice.
Then gathered in a circle
    To hear coach give some advice.

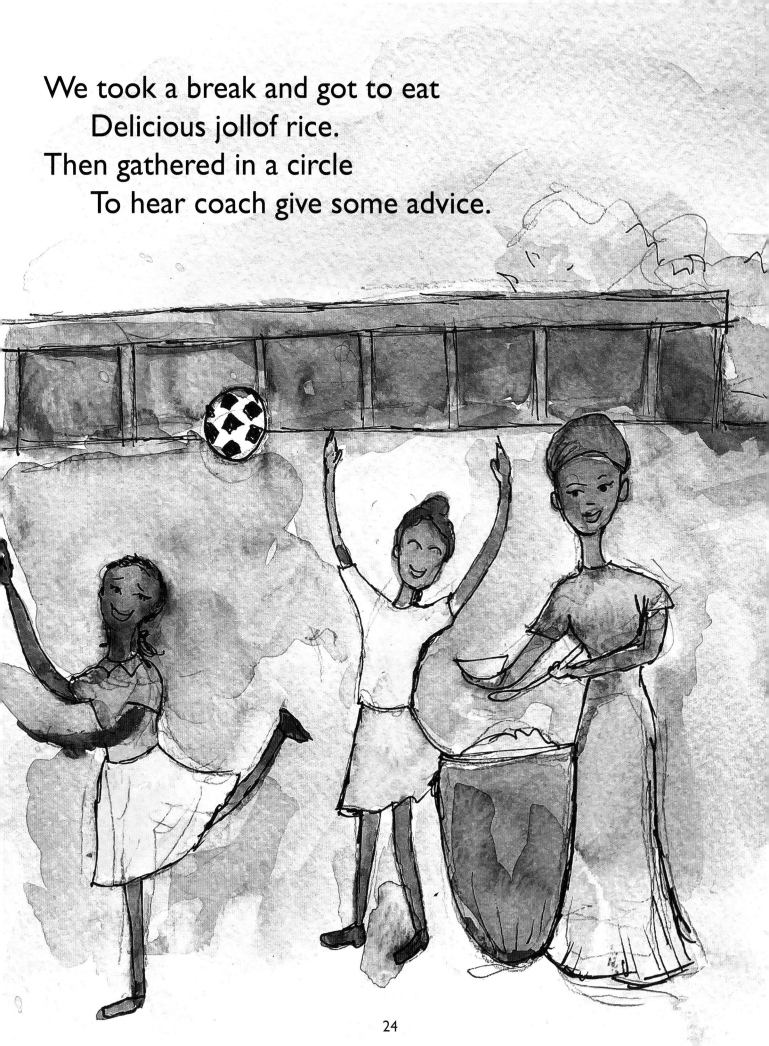

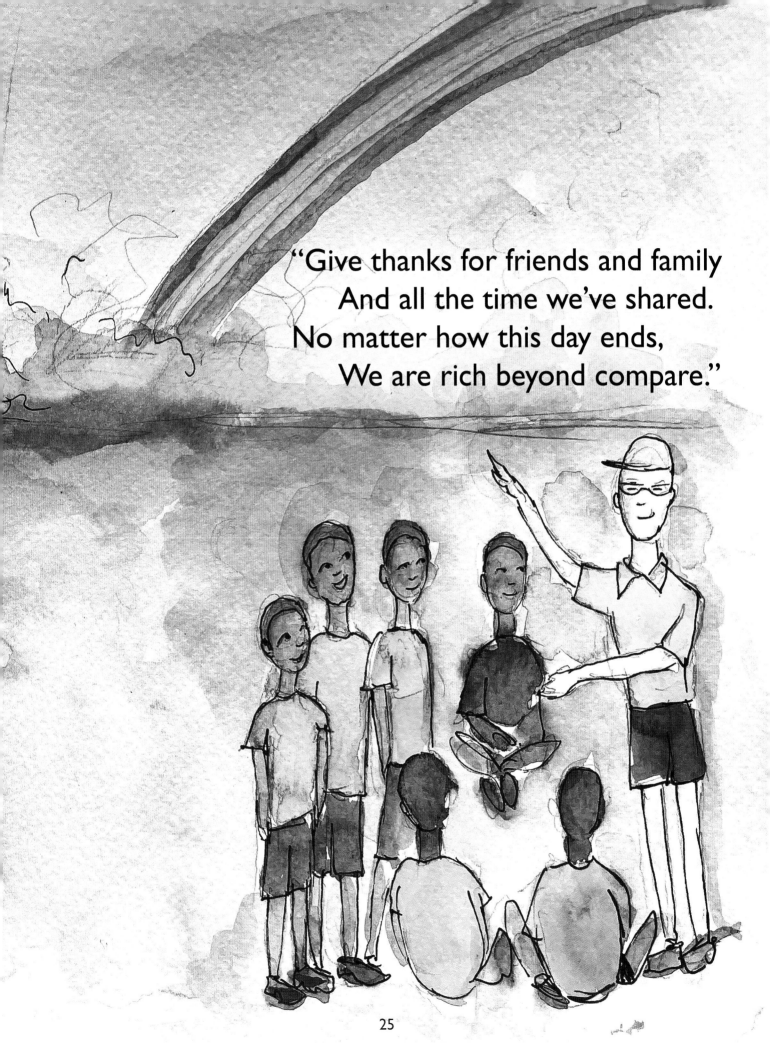

"Give thanks for friends and family
And all the time we've shared.
No matter how this day ends,
We are rich beyond compare."

And then we played the last game.
    In the end the score was tied.
The sun was slowly setting…
    And we all were very tired.

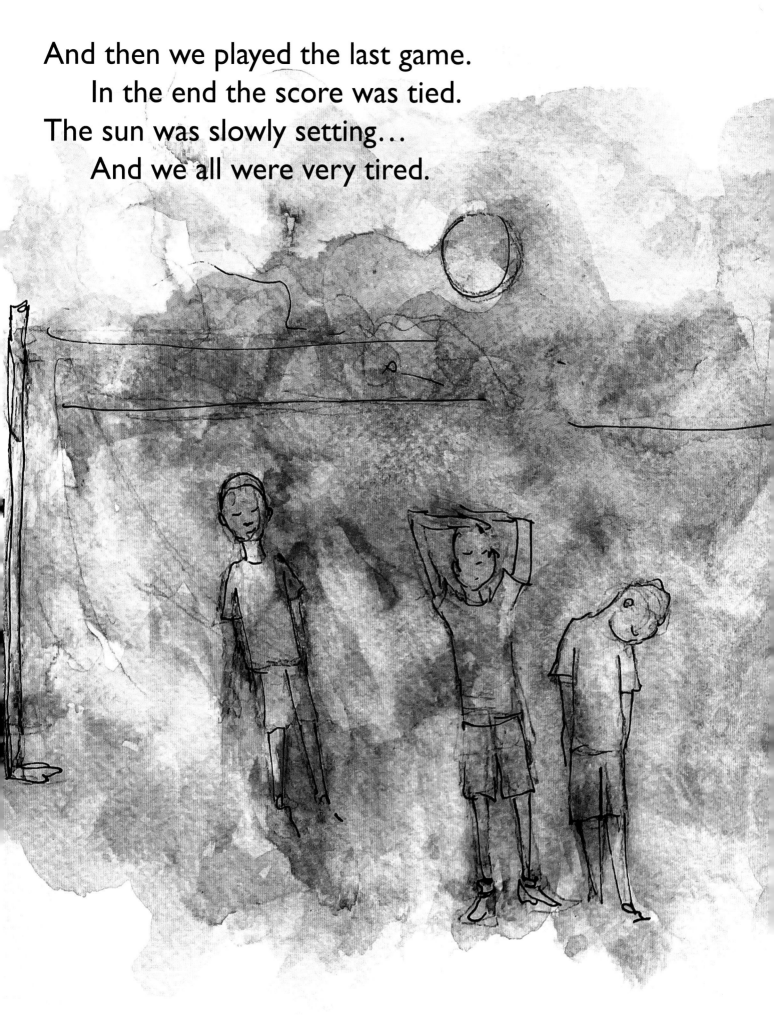

So, who would win the tournament?
You can't just tie the score.
There had to be a champion
And so we played some more.

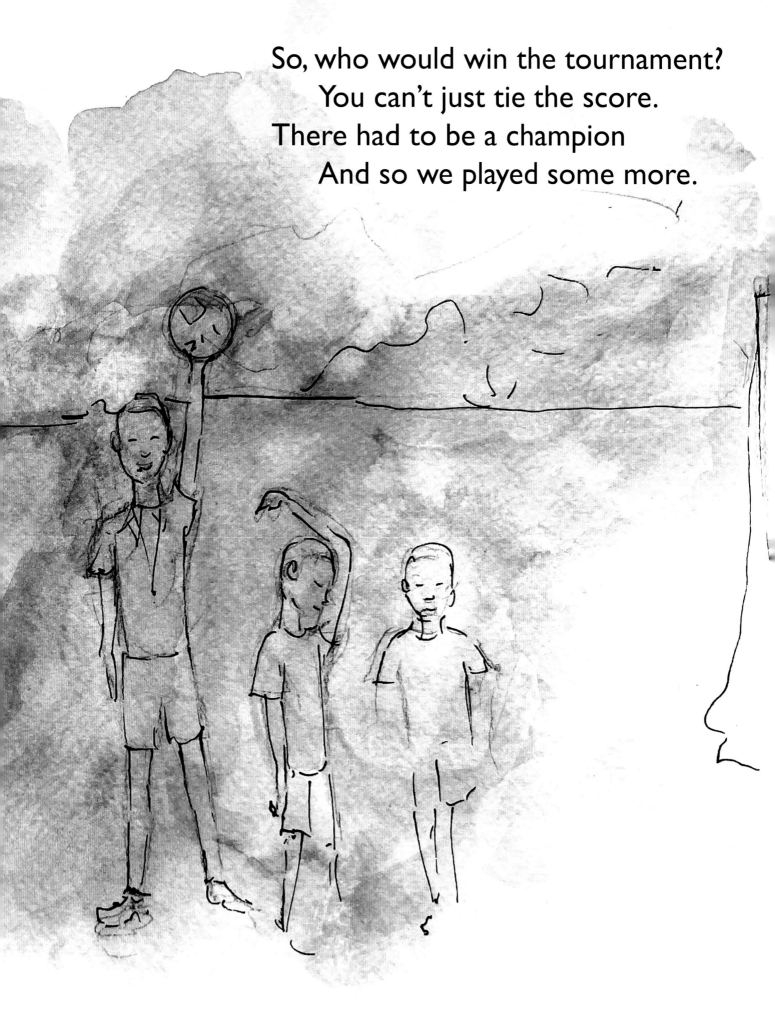

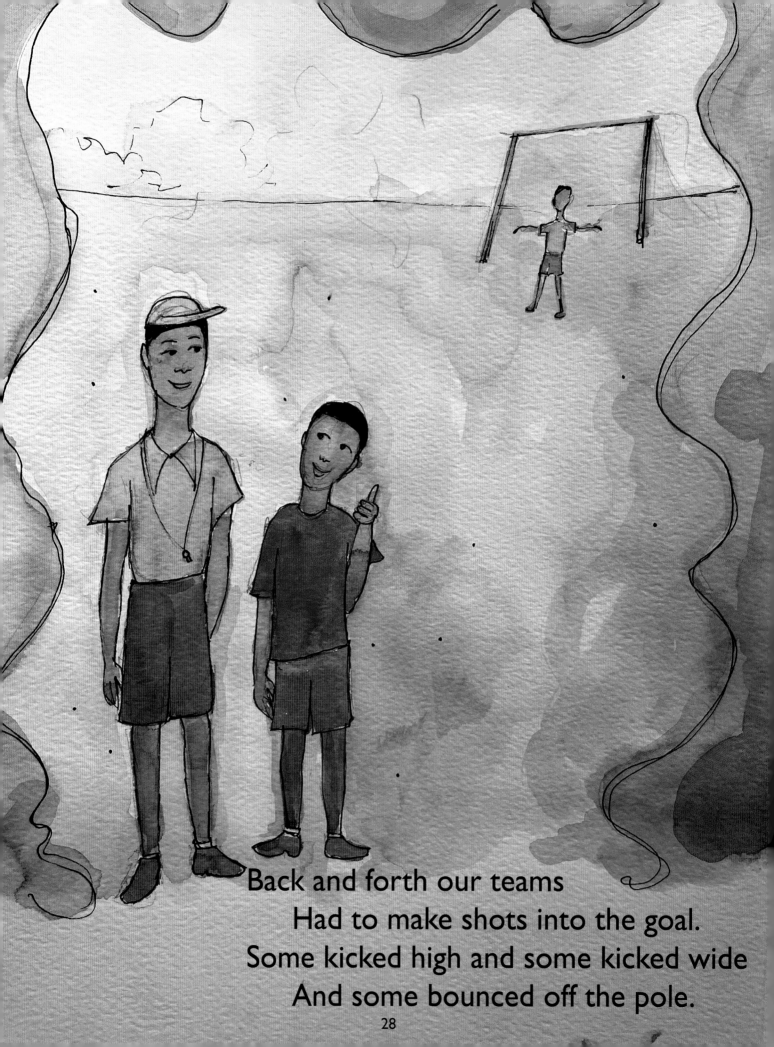

Back and forth our teams
　　Had to make shots into the goal.
Some kicked high and some kicked wide
　　And some bounced off the pole.

Just like in practice, we would win
    If I kicked in the net.
I started running forward once my
    Plan was good and set.

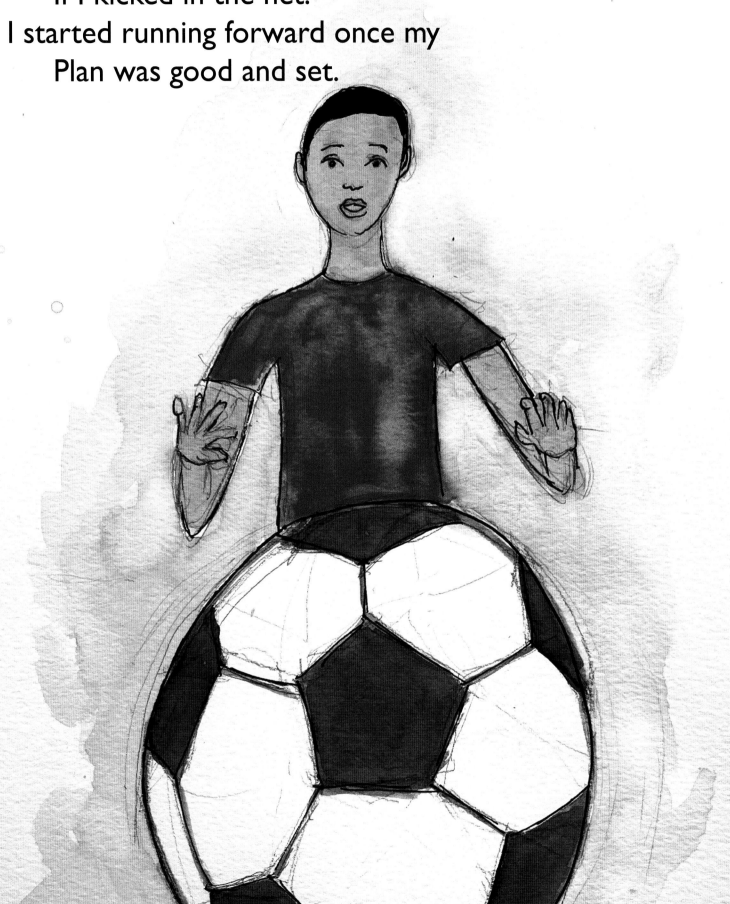

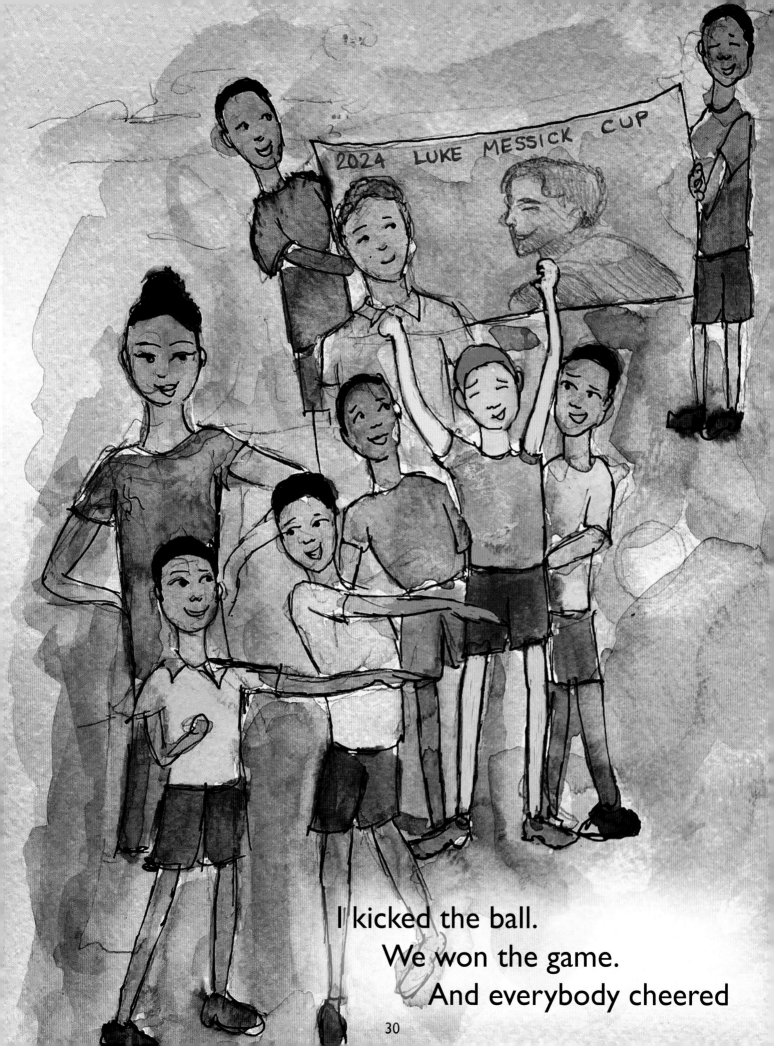

I kicked the ball.
We won the game.
And everybody cheered

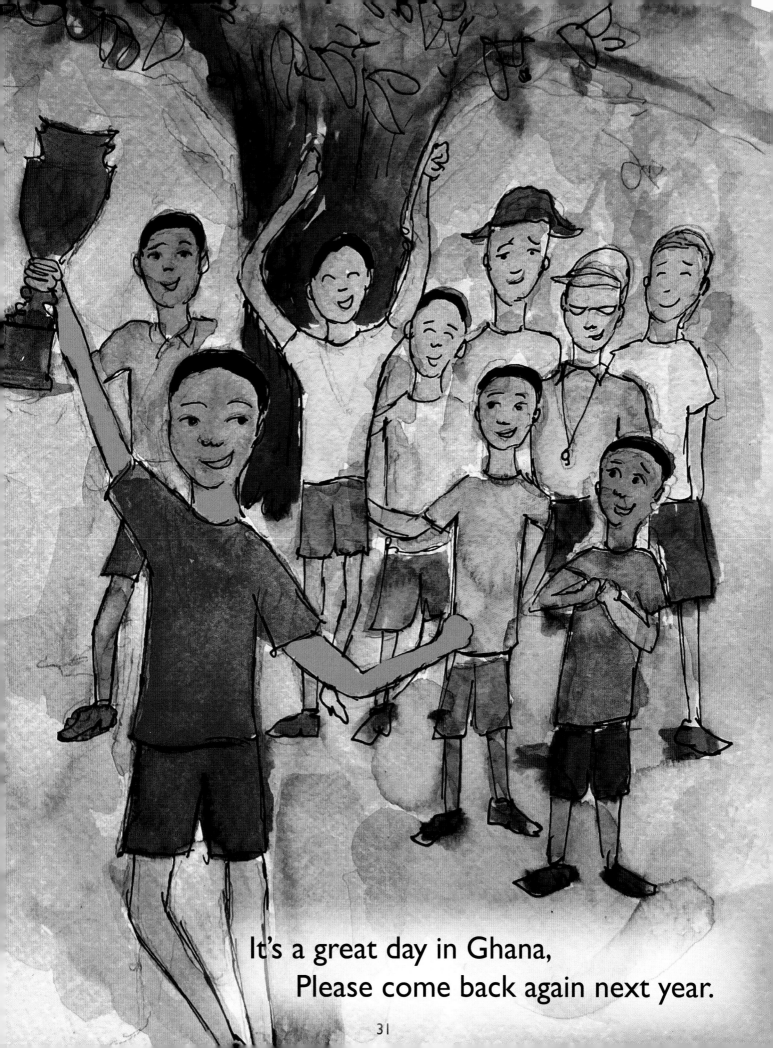

It's a great day in Ghana,
Please come back again next year.

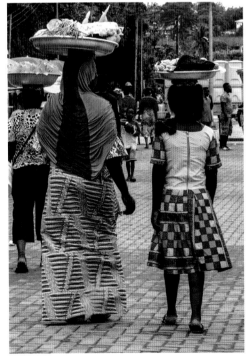

Coaches Isaac, Joshua, Emmanuel, and Alex with members of the Ghana National Team.

Shutterstock

# About Ghana

The story you just read is based on true experiences of players and coaches in Ghana. The country is located on the mid-western side of Africa. The children in this book live in Accra, which is the capital of Ghana.

As you may have noticed, many families in Ghana have chickens to provide eggs for their family. It is not unusual to see these chickens running freely through communities, along with goats that provide milk.

Small shops line the streets of Accra providing food, clothes, and other supplies. Traffic can get busy in the capital city and there are many traffic jams. Thankfully, there are vendors who walk past the stopped cars selling almost anything you might need. Ice cold water, matches to light your home stove, hard-boiled eggs, peanuts, plantains, and so much more. The sales people balance their products right on top of their heads!

English is the official language of Ghana, which makes travel by Americans especially easy. The team is led by a group of men who once played on the same school field. The players are local children, including orphans, who live nearby.

Salespeople carry goods on their heads in Ghana. (ROSN123 - Shutterstock)

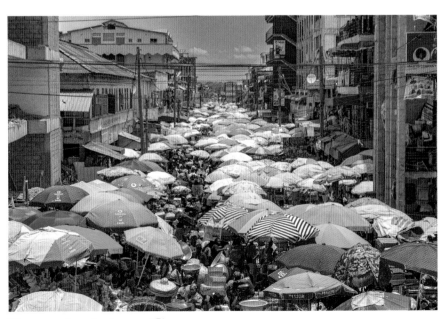

The market in Accra, Ghana. (Omri Eliyahu - Shutterstock)

# About Luke

A chance discovery on Instagram connected Virginia soccer goalie Luke Messick with young soccer players in Accra, Ghana. Noticing that the players had lots of spirit but lacked shoes and other equipment, Luke was able to get his friends in the United States to donate supplies and funds which were sent to Africa.

Luke's plans for Ghana did not end when he was killed by a distracted driver speeding down the highway. Instead, Luke's family and friends across the soccer community created Luke Messick Futbol Charities, Inc. The non-profit group has sent hundreds of pounds of shoes and supplies to Ghana. In addition, they have sponsored soccer tournaments in Virginia, provided college scholarships, sent deserving children to summer soccer camps, and repaired and built safe facilities for the players in Ghana.

At home and abroad, Luke brought energy to every team he played… winning the prestigious Golden Gloves award at the North American Sand Soccer Championships. Most of all, he brought his love of the game to others… even those who were half way around the world. Visit www.lukemessickfc.com to learn more.

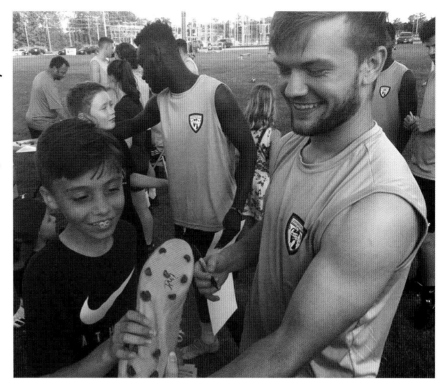

*Luke signs a shoe for a fan. (Lionsbridge FC)*

*Coaches Shaw and Caeman prepare shoes and shirts for Ghana. 99-year-old Jeanne Kent helps!*

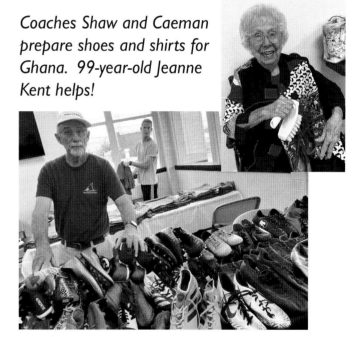

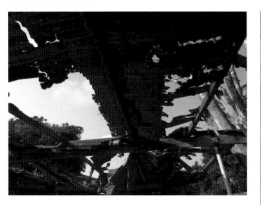
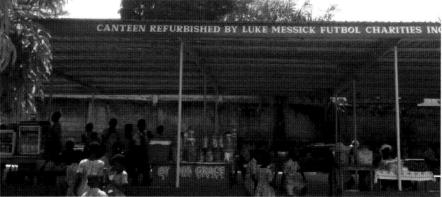

*The canteen (before and after repairs) is where students and players eat lunch and escape the heat.*

# Coach Shaw and the Team

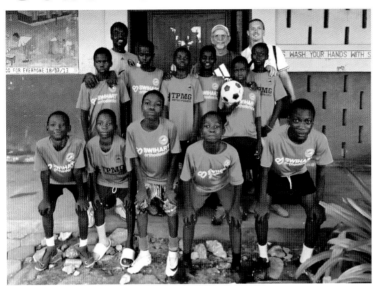

*The winning team with Coaches Isaac, Shaw, and Joshua.*

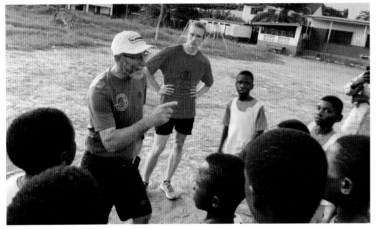

*Coach Shaw and Joshua with the team.*

Steve Shaw is a professional soccer player, coach, and instructor. Luke Messick was one of many players who benefited from his training. When the decision was made to send soccer coaches to Ghana, Steve was the first person asked and he said "yes" right away.

He has participated in mission trips to China where he taught English and helped small villages construct bridges. He has visited Africa several times, providing his coaching expertise and bringing much needed equipment.

As coach of the Christopher Newport University Soccer Team from 1996 to 2018, Steve Shaw's team became the first CNU sport to earn a number one national ranking. He also led the team to four National Quarterfinals and five conference tournament titles.

Luke's brother Joshua and his two college roommates, Liam and Caeman, have also been part of the mission and have provided training in Africa.

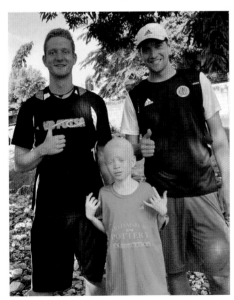

*Coach Caeman and Coach Liam with Christopher.*

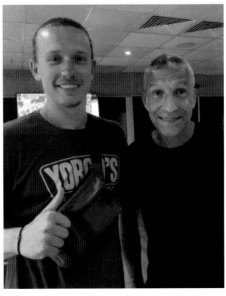

*Joshua with Ghana National Team Coach Chris Houghton.*

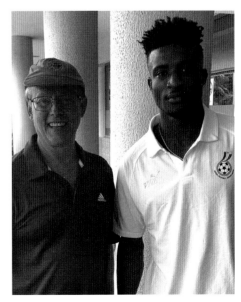

*David with Soccer Superstar Mohammed Kudus.*

# Things to Consider

There is a lot to be learned about Ghana in this book. Some can be found in the words… some in the pictures.

- How is the school in Ghana like your school? How is it different?
- How is the market in Ghana like markets you've visited? How is it different?
- Is the soccer field in Ghana like any you have seen? How is it different?
- What made Coach Shaw and his team, "rich beyond compare?"
- For what are you thankful?
- What do you love to do?
- How can you share what you love to do with others?
- Why is practice important?

# Excited about Reading

*(Clockwise) The class is thrilled to get their own books. David shares stories and songs in a classroom. Coach Shaw reads to some of the team members.*

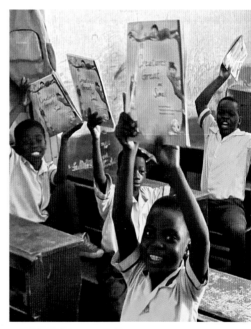

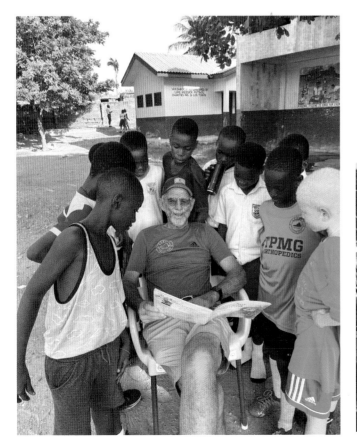

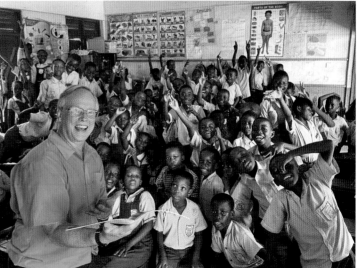

## Books by David Messick, Liu Light, and Cory Steiger

The Amazing Adventures of Chessie the Manatee
Creatures Great and Small
Mary Peake and the Mighty Acorn
The Mother Goose Show
Never Give Up, Short Stories about Big Dreams
Open a Book
The Perilous Predicaments of Pinocchio
The Tall, the Tough, and the Tiny
Virginia Born—Amazing People from the Commonwealth
Virginia Treasures—Amazing Places in the Commonwealth
Wanda's Wondrous Wetland
You Can Do That?  Amazing People with Amazing Jobs

## Audio Programs from David and the Rainbow Puppets

The Amazing Adventures of Chessie the Manatee
From the Sea to the Sky
Jonah
The Mother Goose Travelling Rock and Roll Show
A Pirate Party
The Really Big Dinosaur Show
Toyland!
The Wetland Revue
The Wright Brothers—See Us Fly!

*Available at Amazon.com, RainbowPuppets.com, and DavidMessick.com*

**David Messick** is the founder of Rainbow Productions.  He has written over a dozen children's books and even more children's shows that have been performed at the Smithsonian, New York's American Museum of Natural History, and many other organizations.  He has worked on development projects for the Oprah Winfrey Show and the Disney Channel and has worked with many legendary performers.  He and his wife Marcy were blessed with two amazing boys, Joshua and Luke.  http://davidmessick.com

**Cory Steiger** is a gifted artist. When not creating illustrations for books, he designs and paints sets for musical theater productions.  He has provided voices for many memorable Rainbow Puppet characters including Rumpelstiltskin and the Boy Who Cried Wolf.  He is currently working on his Masters of Fine Art in Set Design at Temple University. And if that weren't enough, he's a Board-Certified Behavior Analyst working to help children.